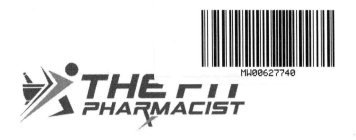

MW00627740

The Pharmacist's Survival Guide

for

Managing Stress

&

Fitting in Fitness

Dr. Adam Martin

How to Become The Fit Pharmacist

All rights reserved. No part of this publication may be reproduced, distributed or transmitted in any form or by any means, including photocopying, recording, or other electronic or mechanical methods, without the prior written permission of the publisher, except in the case of brief quotations embodied in critical reviews and certain other noncommercial uses permitted by copyright law.

Table of Contents

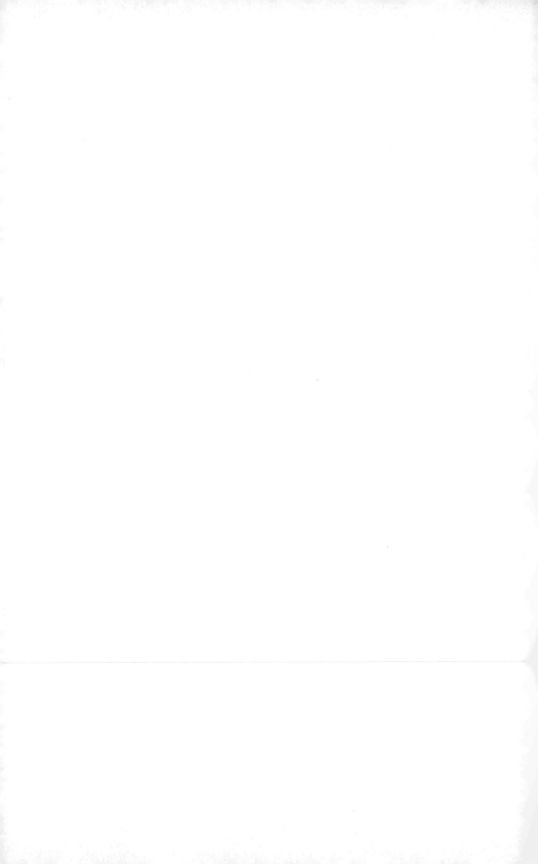

How to Become The Fit Pharmacist

*Simple Solutions for the Pharmacist
to Master Your Mindset,
Nail Your Nutrition, and
Fit in Fitness*

I. ℞: The Why Behind This Book

My name is Dr. Adam Martin, and I am the founder of The Fit Pharmacist. When I was in pharmacy school, I noticed something profound in all of my classes: **Nutrition** is the cornerstone of therapy for literally every single disease state we help to treat as healthcare professionals, *yet we are not given much training as to the science behind it*. Patients will come to you very frequently asking questions related to nutrition- what are you going to say? If you *do* know some answers, are YOU using those tips yourself? Are you leading them to better health through your own example to inspire their journey?

In healthcare, we strive every day to improve the lives of those that we serve. Sometimes we can care so deeply and give so much, that we do so for the *sacrifice of our own health*. At first it starts small- skipping a meal, forgoing that one workout- but over time, it can become a habit that forms an unhealthy lifestyle. We can literally fall into the trap of sacrificing our own health thinking it's a dichotomy, that it's just "expected" or "part of the job". I saw this as a student going through pharmacy school, working with extremely passionate healthcare providers who would try things like smoke to curb stress, binge eat after work because they hadn't eaten for 10 hours, or grab anything that was available to munch on (which more often than not was some of the unhealthiest food options you can imagine). I started to see this more and more, even as I graduated and became a full-time pharmacist living that high workload lifestyle, and I thought to myself: ***there's GOT to be a better way!***

How can we, as healthcare providers, not live up to the standard that we ourselves are preaching to our patients on improving their own health? I wanted to be an example for patients, friends and family, someone who can empower them and support them through their own journey into living their best lives. Not stopping at my role as a pharmacist, but to be more, to live a healthy lifestyle *myself* that is practical, realistic, and simple- so simple that ANY healthcare professional could do it- without having to follow a restrictive meal plan or rely on expensive supplements.

For me to be able to truly grasp this as a healthcare provider feels like a gift I need to share, so that others can become empowered and live life on their own terms, feeling AMAZING and actually enjoying the process along the way! To me, being a pharmacist is one of the most special things in my life – the relationships I form with my colleagues and patients through that trust is truly sacred. But being able to go even deeper, and being able to help people through nutrition is INDESCRIBABLE- allowing them to really understand how to eat for their own goals by simplifying the science - it's really hard to put that feeling of impact into words, honestly!

I want YOU to be able to thrive for the rest of your lives, to become YOUR own best nutritionist – to have that knowledge to be able to be at any pharmacy, hospital, medical school - anywhere in the world - and be able to successfully achieve YOUR goals with ease using the SimpleSolutions outlined in this book. My goal is to take the frustration out of what healthy living as a healthcare practitioner does NOT have to be! To have us be in total control over what's going on in our body.

You don't have to be a pharmacist, a nutritionist, or anyone other than yourself- with a genuine desire to live life on your terms by controlling the controllables, through these SimpleSolutions that will without a doubt allow you to script your own success so that you can live your ideal life of health. And THAT is what healthcare is all about- caring enough to lead others to optimal health.

Disclaimer

All of the information presented in this text is for educational and resource purposes only. It is there to help you make informed decisions about health-related fitness issues. It is not a substitute for any advice given to you by your physician. Always consult your physician or health care provider before beginning any nutrition or exercise program. Use of the programs, advice, and information contained in this text is at the sole choice and risk of the reader. You are solely responsible for the way you perceive and utilize information in this text and you do so at your own risk. In no way will Adam Martin, Kori Propst, or any persons and or entities associated with The Fit Pharmacist, LLC be held responsible for any injuries or problems that may occur due to the use of this text or the advice contained therein. Prior to beginning any physical fitness regimen or making any nutritional changes you are strongly urged to consult your physician. In addition, none of the information in this book should be taken as legal or financial advice. Always ensure to adhere to state and federal laws when practicing pharmacy and specific policies and procedures that are required by your employer.

II. ℞: Introducing the Need for Health in Healthcare

Go to the gym. Eat healthy. Sounds like a simple plan, right? If you are looking to live life as a healthy healthcare professional, there is something you may have picked up on: *simple does not mean easy*.

Take the pharmacy manager who works the standard 40-hour workweek- PLUS picks up extra hours if they're offered- PLUS gets to work early and stays late- PLUS has a family of 4 that needs provided for- PLUS has to handle the mortgage, the family car and all of its maintenance, making sure the kids do their homework, go grocery shopping, have a social life, attend family gatherings, plan vacation... where and when does taking care of yourself fit?

Or the pharmacist who works full-time, has an hour-long commute one-way, newly married, a kid on the way, trying to close on a home, taking care of his elderly parents, helping the wife find a new job, looking for a new church, and is managing his brother's finances. Is it even possible to THINK about being healthy?

While many of us have fallen prey to the feeling "I don't have time" or "I can't afford to spend time on my own health", I beg you to consider the exact opposite: **you can't afford NOT to!** Imagine what would happen to your ever-so-carefully planned balancing act if you get to spend a month in the hospital because you decided to ignore your slowly rising weight gain, the shortness of breath that progressed, or other red flag warnings the body is trying to get your attention with that you need to pay attention here and take care of yourself!

"Yes, but…"

If that's what immediately comes to mind, I am not judging you! In fact, I am willing to bet that you feel you are sacrificing your own "me" time for the sake of giving to others more. Choosing to spend your time for others rather than yourself. A selfless act of love. If you take this too far, it in fact becomes *selfish*! I am NOT telling you to live in the gym or advising you to go work on a nutrition degree. That, too, would potentially be selfish! And probably unrealistic, especially in the above scenarios or our own life situation.

Why?

Aint' nobody got time fo dat!

Either extreme can prove detrimental to both your health and the health of those you love. So what are we to do?! Not prioritizing health leads us to the hospital, yet becoming a fitness fanatic leaves us feeling selfish and even neglectful of those we love? Can we ever win?! Yes, yes we can! Yes, yes YOU can. Some of the most common barriers I have heard from pharmacists who genuinely *want* to be healthier, but feel that they can't, may sound familiar to you as well:

"I don't have enough time."

"I hate the gym- it's so intimidating!"

"I eat healthy, but I don't lose any weight! I have even GAINED some and I watch what I eat!"

"I don't even get a lunch break- how am I supposed to even CONSIDER eating healthy as a pharmacist?! It's not realistic!!"

"It's just so complicated with my work schedule!"

"Eating healthy is so expensive- I can't afford it!"

"Nutrition, working out- it's all so overwhelming! I don't know where to start- there's so much conflicting information about what works!"

No, I'm not going to cut to an infomercial for an overpriced magic shake or some super fancy workout equipment that has been approved by NASA and the NIH- I'm not here to sell you anything. What I am here to do is offer you some SimpleSolutions to life's seemingly most complex, frustrating, and overwhelming barriers to HOW you can realistically fit in fitness into your daily life- mental, nutritional, and physical fitness. The most common block people have, *"I don't have time"*, is something I do want to address right now. It's not that you don't have time- it's that you don't have a realistic plan that will work with your current lifestyle...*yet*. Practicality and efficiency are the characteristics that you will find with each and every tip within this book, because simple works! Simple we can do! Simple will lead us from day one, to day two, to day three- and this will build consistency. Compound consistency over time and what do you get? RESULTS! That is what I hope to share with you all in the coming pages as we take the guesswork out of how to live a healthy life, and offer SimpleSolutions to empower you to build momentum, which you can then scale into creating your ideal health, however that looks – or feels- to you! Let's begin:

III. ℞: MASTER YOUR MINDSET

"What the mind believes, the body achieves"

Who better a professional to start us off on THE most important aspect of healthy living than my good friend and world-leading expert Dr. Kori Propst! Here is a little about why what she is about to tell you matters- A LOT- and how her wisdom and guidance will empower you to start living your best life where all of your actions stem from: your mind!

The
Diet Doc
Feel the Change

Dr. Kori Propst is the Wellness Director and Vice President of The Diet Doc, LLC. Licensed in Clinical Mental Health Counseling and a Licensed Professional Counselor, Kori has earned a bachelor's degree in exercise physiology, a master of science in counseling, and a doctorate in health psychology and behavioral medicine. Her dissertation addressed the perceived threats to weight loss goals and their relationship to motivation and Self-Determination. Her education is enhanced by certifications in personal training, health coaching, and lifestyle

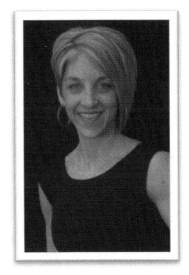

and weight-management consulting. She is an ISSN (International Society of Sports Nutrition) clinician.

The Diet Doc specializes in educational consulting for individuals who desire to achieve optimal *and sustainable* health.

She uses experiential approaches to move her clients from chaos to capacity. They glean insight into their strengths and apply them toward optimizing their potentials! When 98% of individuals who lose weight gain it back, it's proof that a cookie-cutter, one-size-fits all approach is ineffective. The Diet Doc's lifestyle based programming encourages individuals to adopt an approach of structured flexibility. With encouragement and the science of motivation built into every step of the process, clients adapt their behaviors and mindsets to facilitate safe, effective, and enduring health practices. Their individual metabolisms, lifestyles, food preferences, health conditions, activity levels, goals, and daily schedules are keys to developing their personal plans for success that can stand the test of time.

Kori specializes in a blend of coaching and therapeutic modalities, including cognitive behavioral, positive psychology, mindfulness, and strengths-based experiential techniques, all geared toward integrative self-determination. Her expertise includes physical and mental training and mind-body integration, optimal performance, and overall well-being.

Kori welcomes any inquiries and can be reached via email at kori@thedietdoc.com.

MASTER YOUR MINDSET ~ Kori Propst, PhD
The 4 A's of Mindset

Attitude
Attitude is the way you dedicate yourself to the way you think.

We all have tendencies and patterns in terms of the way we think, but I want you to remember something. Tendencies need not become actualities. We are our energy governors. What we focus on grows. Where our focus goes, energy flows! So you tell me, if you think in a negative way, what are the consequences?

What happens when you adopt a curious mindset versus a catastrophic mindset?
A black and white attitude versus a neutral attitude?

When you say "I can" versus "I can't," and even better ask, "how can I?" what happens to the energy within you? Curiosity opens you up, right? We expand into the possibilities versus close down and contract.

As you move into the situations of your lives begin the practice of asking, "What attitude am I choosing?" Notice right now what attitude you are choosing as you read this book. What attitude will you choose as you engage in conversations with your peers? What attitude will you choose when your head hits the pillow tonight, and when your feet hit the floor in the morning?

You can choose an attitude of determination, an attitude of zest, an attitude of compassion, an attitude of assertiveness, an attitude of wonder, an attitude of gratitude, an attitude of patience, an attitude of enthusiasm, an attitude of love, an attitude of perspective. And remember, your attitude can change minute to minute if you want it to. That's up to you!

Attention
Attention is a type of awareness. To understand attention, we can ask ourselves "What am I paying attention to?"

At any one time, our attention is on *something.* We may be in the middle of a conversation with someone and our attention is not at all on what the person is saying. Instead, our attention may be on what our next meal is going to be...or even how we want to respond to the person we're speaking with.

Another way to think about attention is by asking, "Where am I allowing my attention to land?"

We have a food diet, for example. This is what we consume in the form of macronutrients, right? But we also have a thought diet—what we consume that directly shapes the manner in which we think, feel, and behave.

Where we let our attention land influences how we perceive the world. If I'm constantly looking at pictures of other athletes and comparing myself to them, I'm choosing where my attention is going.

A reflection for you: is what you are paying attention to, in your service?

Go back to the first A. What attitude does it prompt for you? Is what you are paying attention to energizing or mentally discouraging? Do you feel the energy in your body collapse or expand?

Finally, it's important to ask, "How am I paying attention?" This question brings us to the quality of attention.

Do I eat and just eat?
Do I listen and just listen in a conversation?
Do I write an email and just concentrate on the email?

Mastering our mindsets means developing a high *quality* attention. I'll repeat the 3 questions you can use to practice this and become more aware of your attention:

1. What am I paying attention to in the moment?

2. Where do I let my attention land (literally, what do you spend your time attending to?)

3. How am I paying attention? (What is the quality of my attention? Is it diffuse or targeted on just one thing?)

Attribution

Attribution is how we ascribe meaning to the circumstances, events, outcomes, and situations of our lives.

Say you get done reading this section of the book, and you're super excited to share what you have learned with your partner! You explain what you've just found out about attitude! You have never thought about the definition of the word, and you have a new understanding of it. You ask your partner about their attitude—what attitude do they notice they bring to conversations with you? Your partner is quiet.

Do you attribute that pause as an indication that your question was stupid and silly?

Does the pause mean nothing to you at all?

Do you attribute the pause to your partner's thoughtfulness and care in wanting to craft the best reply?

Do you attribute the pause to the possible waft of cold air your partner felt from the sea breeze that just came through the window?

You get my point.

Or let's say that you miss your lift at your next meet...or you stumble over your words as you give a presentation to your colleagues.

Do you attribute the event to your worth as a human being? "I don't know what I thought I could do that well anyway..."

Or do you attribute it to needing more practice, so you go home and watch the video you recorded and assess it both for what you did well and then what you could improve upon?

Attribution is related to our worldviews and whether we have an internal locus of control or an external locus of control.

Do we take compassionate responsibility or do we place blame on others or things?

When we place blame, there's nothing we can do about it, right? We are left stuck. The consensus is that we are who we are and we can't grow.

Dr. Carol Dweck, who researches intelligence, brilliantly articulates the differences in individuals who operate with a fixed or growth mindset. Those with a fixed mindset attribute difficulty, hardship, or mistakes to a lack of intelligence. "I am the way I am."

On the other hand, those with a growth mindset understand that intelligence is built, incrementally, and attributed to effort and practice.

Your reflection question for attribution is as follows:

What are all the contributing factors associated with this outcome? (This assumes you will be finding both internal and external influences, which is a healthy manner of assuming responsibility and solution-solving).

Agility

Perhaps you've heard the term "behavioral flexibility." I know you've heard the term "structured flexibility" if you are familiar with The Diet Doc's method of sustainable nutrition!

I like to use the term agility as it pertains to mindset mastery because it conveys coordination, quickness, alertness, and an ability to shift easily.

An agile mindset is one that views "hard" differently.

Imagine having an attitude of enthusiasm for hard versus an attitude of discouragement because you didn't get something "right" the first time. When I started road cycling I had to learn how to clip in and out of my pedals. I fell multiple times and I have the scars to prove it. Each time I fell I asked myself what I could learn and how I could do it differently the next time. With each bruise and scrape I became *more* engaged! I could say, "this is *hard!*" with excitement and a little less frustration.

HARD is Harnessing Awareness, Resilience, and Determination.

Do you have an agile mindset that views hard in that way? A mindset that can switch easily from assertive to vulnerable, to compassionate, to curious, to appreciative, to zestful?

The question that can open you up to develop your mindset agility is this:

What is one action I might take to approach this situation as an opportunity?

An agile mind is set toward "leaning in" when discomfort arises; viewing the difficult as a challenge rather than a threat; and doing a backbend over a barrier rather than avoiding it!

You have the capacity within you to achieve your most lofty goal pursuits. One thing I might add that can accelerate your process is to align with others. Find a community in which to live into your questions and learn together. In doing so, you not only gather new ideas and perceptions and step out of your box, but you also have the opportunity to contribute. We know that contributing to the betterment of others creates more positive emotions and engagement! The Fit Pharmacist community is an excellent option in this regard ☺

Emotional Eating

Emotional eating is all about how we relate to the thoughts in our minds...and the energies in our bodies.

Emotions are energy in motion. That's it. When something occurs within the environment that shifts our experience, our energy changes. You *feel* these shifts all the time. No doubt, you notice when you experience a wave of fatigue. Energy shift. You notice when you experience a lack of focus or clarity. Energy shift. You notice when you experience a sense of heaviness. Energy shift.

Now, the *feeling* is what you label the energy shift. Using the examples above, the feelings would be *tired, stressed, and discouraged,* respectively.

It's not the emotion that causes us to eat. Energy is just energy. What moves us toward food is the how we view the label we give the emotion.

Let's use the experience of stress as an example. If I have an experience of shifting focus, and I have the thought, "Man, I can't concentrate. I'm so freaking stressed," there is a tone of disdain and negativity attached, right? I'm looking at the feeling as bad...as one I perhaps *shouldn't* be having. In this case, I perceive the feeling as threatening. In other words, it's harmful to my sense of well-being and balance. So what do I do? I aim to change it, stop it, or get away from it. Where's the vending machine?

Here's the problem with this perceived "solution": it doesn't work long-term. Food may momentarily distract us, however, when emotions are there, they're there. They aren't going anywhere unless we acknowledge them or give them time to work through. And work through they will, if we don't try to stuff them away. Because they are energy, they move, and research shows they take about 30-60 seconds to pass by.

So rather than attempting to eat them away or use food to *feel* better, how about we learn to feel *better*? What a novel concept, right? We're human and we'll have shifts in energy influenced by relationships, the environment, the circumstances of our lives because that's literally how we human, so let's learn to human *better!*

How to Human Better (Instead of Emotionally Eating)

Practice becoming the observer of the experience you're having. Pretend you are a fly on the wall of your internal living space. When an energy shift occurs, try saying, "Hmm...that's an interesting change" and then begin putting your focus on the sensations (root word **senses**). Notice whether there is heat or cold, tightness, laxity, aching, pressure, heaviness, or speed anywhere within you...or even outside of you. In this way you are taking note of the emotional charge in your body. But you're not judging what you notice—you are just observing. Do this with sight, sound, touch, taste, and smell as well. In so doing, you are refocusing your attention to become grounded. What often happens is that we'll become snagged by the "definition" of the experience and then begin telling a story about it that turns into the disaster that we need to get out of immediately!

The story I've mentioned above is the thought stream inside our minds. We have thousands of thoughts a day, most of which are just random, mean nothing, and carry little weight. Until they do...because we've decided to engage with them and view them as directives. We need to learn to relate to our thoughts differently. What I see most people do is to try to not have any thoughts, stop the thoughts they do have, or immediately try to change the thought. But the harder you try to get rid of a thought or not think about something, the more you'll think about it. You're focused on it! This is called the **Ironic Process Theory**. A more optimal strategy is again, to practice becoming an observer. This time, you become an observer of your mind. When a thought pops up, you might say, "Oh, ha. Hi there. You're interesting. We could spin a mighty tale, but I think I'll just let you ride on by..." You might imagine a thought bubble with the words inside of it. You see the bubble. You pop the bubble. The words disperse. You refocus your attention. Ever laid on the ground and just watched the clouds in the sky? Some float by, others stick around a bit longer but lumber along, many are wispy and leave remnants but then eventually disappear? Our thoughts are the same. I also imagine thoughts as brain burps. When we burp, what do we do? We acknowledge the burp (if we're civilized humans) by saying "excuse me!" and then we move on, usually never thinking about the burp again, right? We can learn to view the thoughts in our minds in the same way.

Now, doesn't eating in times of emotion sound silly? Emotions are temporary. So is the satisfaction or distraction we feel when we eat to get away from them. Only, eating piles on a whole host of other issues. Learning to human and have energy moves us out of emotional eating to emotional intelligence!

4 Methods for Mastering Stress & Overwhelm
All of you have goals that you are striving to pursue with the greatest level of consistency, tenacity, and motivation as possible, right?

You want to avoid making mistakes, and yet you know they are inevitable.

So what do we do when we find ourselves mired in negative thinking, self-doubt, contemplating giving up, or even just wondering what we can do to shift into a better space when your mojo feels like it has disappeared?

First, let's define mastery. After all, it's what all of you are interested in becoming...masters of your mindset, masters of your craft, and masters of your goals. So what does mastery mean?

Mastery is *not* "meeting the goal." Because as all of you have encountered, there's the question of "now what?" As humans when we accomplish something, we move on pretty quickly! Okay....next!

So if we know this, and we want to pursue our goals with heightened and sustained motivation, then we have to look at mastery not as an outcome, but as a process.

Mastery is:

Expansion of your vision
Development of character
Stepping into opportunities
Carving out your path to your potential
Adapting to grow into an integrated identity
Stretching from your current capacities into the future possibilities

Here is what I'm proposing—that no matter what your goal, you will avoid losing your mind if you approach *whatever* you do as a practice in becoming a pretty cool human.

I think if we focus on becoming a human of integrity, *not* losing our minds becomes a bit easier. Our focus, as Sarah Lewis has been quoted as saying, is that "mastery is in the reaching, not the arriving."

So mastery is a process of reaching...of becoming. So let's talk about *how* we can practice mastery. I'll give you four ways!

Practice #1 for *not* losing your mind is this: Practice! **Utilize your life as a practice ground!**

Wait, what?! Yep, we get to approach everything we do—*life!*—as our classroom. As I'm sharing this information with you, I'm practicing articulating information in such a way that is understandable. I'm practicing not getting lost in my own thoughts and allowing the material to flow organically! I'm practicing a bit of storytelling as examples to bring the information to life!

When something happens in our lives that we don't like, viewing the event as an opportunity for practicing a more effective response can help us move forward as opposed to feeling stuck.

We can view life as happening *for* us versus *to* us!

When we view life as happening *to* us, we're sucked into a vortex of choicelessness. We feel like we're backed into a corner. And guess what happens when we don't perceive we have any choices? We flip out. We can't concentrate. We either get super rigid and unyielding or we get all chaotic and bent out of shape.

How many of you who are dieting currently have eaten something not on your plan or gone over your macros in some way? Now, when that has happened, what do you do next? Do you freak out a bit and say, "What the hell! I've screwed up the day, so I might as well just eat and start again tomorrow...or the next day...or *Monday!*"?

Or do you crack down on yourself and say, "I'll exercise twice as much tomorrow and not eat any carbs for the day!"?

The first way is chaotic. The second way is rigid.

Either way, you were caught in a space of anxiety and helplessness, and you reacted.

Except you weren't helpless.

More effective choices are always present, if we allow ourselves a pause, a breath (or two or three), and some compassion. We may not like the choices, but that is beside the point. They are there for us to notice.

We can practice pausing and breathing, and then we can practice offering ourselves compassion...all in the name of using this life to practice more powerful, effective responses toward becoming a person of integrity. We view the circumstances as a path to potential.

Now, as athletes and pursuers of fitness goals we may tend toward toughness, right?
Physical toughness—heck yes!
Mental toughness—oh yeah!
We want discipline and regimentation and grit!

Except here's the deal—all of those things are supported by compassion.
Grit is, in fact, *passion* plus persistence, and discipline relies on compassionate energy. Surprised?

Many of you may be thinking that especially when you've let yourself down or engaged in a behavior you're not proud of, that the *best* course of action is to blast yourself with shaming epithets or use harsh language to motivate yourself.

"You're so stupid! I can't believe you did that!" or "What is wrong with you? You really thought you'd get that right?!"

You guys tell me. If your coach, colleague, or friend said that to you, would you feel ignited and enthusiastic? Maybe to punch him in the face!

It's not true that critical self-feedback works as a long-term strategy, and your confidence and self-esteem will *not* grow as a result of doing so.

Because it's *that* important and consequential, your second practice is self-compassion!

Self-Compassion

When you offer yourself compassion it does not mean you're letting yourself off the hook. What you *are* doing is reminding yourself of your humanity—your *common* humanity. We are a part of a larger community of individuals who *all* make mistakes. Yep, we are fallible and in that fallibility incredibly unique and relatable and honestly, more fun.

How many of you want a *perfect* friend? And how many of you would trust a coach to guide you who hadn't him/herself experienced difficulty?

Self-compassion looks like you becoming an advocate for yourself. "Kori, you got this. Kori, hard is fun. Hard is harnessing awareness, resilience, and determination."

Self-compassion engenders responsibility.

Blasting ourselves encourages discouragement and threatens one of our most important psychological needs, **competence**.

Fun fact: research out of Michigan State has revealed that speaking to ourselves in the third person during stressful situations can help us manage emotions more effectively than if we talked to ourselves in the first person.

Say I ended up eating more than I had planned when I went out to dinner with friends. Asking, "Okay, Kori, what one thing about this situation would you choose to influence right now?" (like we're talking *to* a friend) produces less emotion than if I asked myself, "Okay, what is one thing about this situation am I going to influence?"

Why is this? Because we experience a bit of what's called **psychological distancing**, and that has implications for increased self-control. We look at self-control as being something we have to exert a lot of effort to engage, right? The word "control" itself almost conveys struggle. Is self-control…uh…willpower…all about white-knuckling out way back to sanity though?

That leads us to your third practice: This is versus I Am.

This Is versus I Am

If I were to ask you how you know when you're angry, or anxious, or bored, would you have an answer?

If I were a fly on the wall, what would I see on the outside that would indicate you are experiencing one of those emotions?

And if I could zip myself up in your skin (a little weird), what would I experience on the inside?

Those of us who are more successful in navigating difficult emotions have this awareness. We can say, "Yeah, when I'm anxious you'd see me get up often when I'm working and walk back and forth to the kitchen, nibbling a lot. You would probably see me twirling my hair. On the inside my thoughts would be flying at me, my mind would seem scattered. I'd have a hard time concentrating or focusing on one thing for any length of time, and my skin would feel tingly."

But there's a next level awareness here, and it's the ability to notice the experience and then name it. There's a concept in psychology called **name it to tame it**—when we can label the experience of an emotion, we can facilitate it dissipating.

Now, *how* we name it is important. If we say, "I am mad," that doesn't have the same beneficial effect as, "This is an experience of anger."

Let's try it together. "I am mad!" Now pause.

Now, "this is an experience of anger."

The second way is like an observation, right? We have distance between us and the emotion. With the first way it's like we *are* the anger. And in that instance, it's much harder to manage it.

If we *are* the anger, then every cell in our body is the anger.

But if this is an experience of anger, is all of me angry or just a part of me?

What we have here is a strategy for practicing becoming the observer of the thoughts and emotions that we experience. We can learn to watch them like a movie as opposed to staring *in* the movie!

And that, my friends, brings us to your fourth practice: become an observer of your mind.

The thoughts we experience are things...just like the chair you're sitting in and the nose on your face. Thoughts are strings of words...until we take the thought a step further and attach a meaning to it.

We can practice watching the thoughts that run across the mind just like they're scrolling on a marquee. Just like they are clouds moving across the sky. Some move fast, some saunter. Some are large and billowing. Others are so wispy we barely notice they're there.

We have thousands of thoughts a day, and most we aren't even aware of. Those that do snag us though, we have an opportunity to practice approaching in a new way. Like someone we're meeting for the first time, for example. We don't know them, we've never seen them. They're interesting!

How might you change if you approached your thoughts with curiosity and openness rather than judgment?

Let's take a thought like, "I want cake!" When you notice that thought do you laugh? Do you talk back to it? "Of course you feel like you want cake. Your family had cake every night after dinner!"

Or do you view it as a directive, your next thought being, "I want cake, so I am going to go find cake….there's no cake…is there anything else I can eat that's sweet…?"

Or maybe it's not a directive for you; it's an indicator that you don't have any self-control and your next thought is, "What's wrong with me that I have these cravings all the time?!"

Each and every one of the thoughts I just used as examples are opportunities to practice observation. How fun to watch our minds like a movie! *This*, is what **mindfulness** is. It's the practice of non-judgmentally becoming aware of the words on your mind…and not needing to do a single thing with them. How cool a concept is that?!

IV. ℞: NAIL YOUR NUTRITION

6 Simple Steps Pharmacists Can Take To Start Eating Healthier

I know what you're thinking:

"I don't even get a lunch break- how am I supposed to even CONSIDER eating healthy as a pharmacist?! It's not realistic!!"

Oh, really? I beg to differ, so says this pharmacist.

"It's just so complicated with my work schedule!"

Take it from someone who has worked full time in the community setting and maintained a healthy lifestyle for nearly a decade: it CAN be done!

NO- it may not *seem* easy at first, which is why so many people fall off the wagon (or back onto the old wagon of bad habits- which way does the wagon go, again?): there is so much "do this, do that" out there that reading it all leads to confusion, and each one is so complex you feel like you need to be a dietician to make it work!

Now don't get me wrong: I was NOT born a master, nor do I proclaim myself to be perfect! However, along my years in pharmacy world I've picked up some Nutrition Ninja Know-How, and compiled a list of my easiest tips for you to help make eating your way to health as simple as possible- all while being a pharmacist! Let's call it Simple Solutions for Scripting Your Success:

## 1.	Eat foods that you actually like!

Have you ever seen some InstaFamous beach babe/bro who is super ripped, and gives out a free nutrition plan? Tilapia, boiled chicken, raw broccoli for days… oh, the gluttony! It may work to stick to someone *else's* plan that worked for them for a week or so, but after a while it's torture! It's best to lay out a plan including healthy foods you actually enjoy so that you can stick to your plan for the long haul. **Consistency** is the name of the success game, so setting yourself up on a plan you *want* to follow will make that possibility a reality!

2. Prepare your foods ahead of time

Have you ever heard of **bulk cooking**? Literally, it's "cook once and done!" rather than cooking each meal as it comes time to eat. Save yourself time by considering cooking once or twice a week (whichever works best for you and you prefer- this is flexibility at its finest!)- I wrote an entire article all about it that you can read on The Fit Pharmacist website (link will be listed in the "Resources" section at the end of this book). Why prepare meals ahead of time, you may ask? So that your meals are ready to go once it comes time to those 30 seconds between your 5 doctor calls, 8 waiters, drive through complaint and tech who just called off ☺

3. Structure Your Flexibility

In the last tip I mentioned flexibility- this concept is KEY to enabling long-term success with not just your results, but your sanity! Have you ever embarked on the glorious journey of adhering to a meal plan that was so restrictive, you started asking yourself "Well, what CAN I eat?!" Consider the **80/20 rule**: 80% of the foods you eat come from whole, nutritious food sources, while allowing yourself the option to incorporate "fun foods" into the other 20% of your diet. Trust me: knowing that yes, you can have that Twinkie/ice cream/piece of pizza because you planned for it will release you from the feeling of being on a restrictive, deprived existence. It's just more fun with sprinkles in your life, FitPharmFam!

4. Identify Your Go-To Convenience Foods for Backup!

When people hear "convenience foods", they automatically assume that it's unhealthy or loaded with salt and fat. This may hold true sometimes, but NOT always! Believe it or not, there are some excellent healthy convenience foods that you can even buy in your pharmacy! You can learn about how to make simple swaps for the most common foods on my website, www.thefitpharmacist.com, to empower you to pick the healthier option. Also, be sure to check my Instagram, @thefitpharmacist , as I make numerous InfoMemes related to healthy food choices that I think you will find helpful! Some other examples include deli meat, single servings of Greek yogurt, protein bars and shakes- the list is large, and you are in charge! See guys: this CAN be simple, and YES, you CAN do this!

5.   KICS: Keep It Consistent, Silly!

You've probably heard of KISS: Keep It Simple, Silly. Well, just for kicks, I created my very own acronym to highlight the importance that being consistent can have not only on keeping you on track to maintain your success, but to make it as simple as possible! **Willpower**: we all have it, but we only have so much in a day! It's a _limited resource_ so why waste it in trying to decide when to eat?! If you come up with a schedule that works best for you, stick to that! For me, I have a few different ones: my days off, my half days that I work, and my full 13-hour days that I work. Yes, there will be some wiggle room (flexibility), but having a general strategy (structure) will allow you to approach your day with ease because you went into it having a plan. Oh man, it's structured flexibility yet again!

6.   Identify Your Triggers for Hunger

Have you ever eaten to manage your emotions? You know- you weren't really hungry, but the day was just so stressful that when you got home the next thing you knew all of your cupboards were open and you realized your family-sized bag of chips was miraculously empty?

This is known as **emotional eating**, and it is alive and well among us pharmacists- you've probably heard it called "stress eating", and may even have experience with eating out of emotion instead of hunger. You don't have to be a slave to anxiety! You can learn to master your emotions, and even manage emotional eating in the previous section written by health psychologist Dr. Kori Propst, "R$_x$: Master Your Mindset". For even more insight and some simple strategies to put these into practice, there are numerous videos up on our YouTube channel specific to this exact topic (check the "Resources" section at the end of this book).

Some go-to pointers are that when you feel yourself moving towards emotionally-driven eating, to come up with some strategy that works for you to keep your mind off of food. Another tip that works for me personally almost every time: **drink water ASAP!** Fun fact: the brain has a hard time distinguishing thirst from hunger, so while you may *feel* hungry, it could actually be that you're thirsty! Chug a bottle of water, wait 5 minutes, then reassess. This could be your problem solved as simple as glass half-empty/half-full; cheers!

So there you have it, FitPharmFam- 6 simple steps YOU can take to get you started to making your life in ClubPharmacy one of health and wellness! My passion is to help those in the profession to live a life full of health and empowerment, for if WE are functioning at our 100%, we can then deliver better care to our patients, colleagues, and loved ones in our lives. You can be the change you wish to see in pharmacy: it all starts with YOU! I have numerous resources to help you on your journey at www.thefitpharmacist.com

I leave you with this:

"The BEST DIET is NOT always the diet which is the best diet PHYSICALLY, but it's the diet that you can TURN INTO A LIFESTYLE that allows you to lose fat and keep it off because you LEARN how to incorporate ALL FOODS IN HEALTHY MODERATION."
-Dr. Layne Norton

V. ℞: Nutrition 101 – Identify "Macros", the 3 Building Blocks of Nutrition

As one of the most accessible health care providers, our patients come to us seeking advice not only for prescription medication and OTC questions, but also on the big question: *"How do I get healthy?"*

Nutrition is the cornerstone of therapy for literally every single disease state we help to treat as pharmacists, yet we are not given much training as to the science behind it. Patients will come to you very frequently asking questions related to nutrition, and I am here to shed light on the most common questions patients want to know on this topic!

I know what you're thinking: what the heck are these "macros" I keep hearing about? Is this some sort of gimmicky trick? Code name? "Macros" is short for macronutrients, represented by carbohydrates, protein, and fat. See, you have heard of them before! Now that that part of the mystery has been solved, let's take a look at what each macro actually is, and how each can be utilized to help you reach your health and fitness goals!

Carbohydrates

If you're Italian, or love Italian food so much that you basically are Italian, I bet you know some carbs! Pasta, bread, spaghetti, oh my! All of these are prime examples of carbohydrates.

As you may know, carbohydrates are the preferred source of energy for our body and mind. Many diets that praise low carb/ketogenic styles of eating as best for fat loss have given this amazing macro a bad wrap (pun!) BUT have you ever tried this style of eating? Long term? How did you feel? I'm guessing the words "sluggish," "irritable," and "NEVER AGAIN!!!" came to mind. Don't fret, this style of eating is not the end-all be-all. You can have your pasta and burn it off, too! The key here is not to go overboard- keep carbs in, but not in excess.

Protein

You don't have to be a bodybuilder to know and enjoy this macro! Fish, chicken, and turkey are the most common examples of lean protein sources. This macro is composed of amino acids (don't those structures from biochem just flood your mind!), making up our cells and tissues. So, that's a pretty big deal, right? In addition to that, this macro also comprises enzymes: those catalysts for all the fun reactions we had to imprint on our brains for the midterm. You won't ever look at greek yogurt the same.

Knowing that protein is made up of amino acids, and that these are complex molecules, it comes to be that it takes the body some extra time to break them down, as well as more energy to do so. Thus, you use more of the energy you eat to break down what you're eating, so less calories used! Not to mention that this marvelous macro does in fact lead to a greater feeling of satiety (feeling full). Keep in mind, that while it does take the body more energy to break it down, we still have to have a need to use it- meaning, you can't do the Brazilian steakhouse on the daily and not gain weight. Moderation is the key to it all!

So, recap: it digests slower, it requires its own calories to be used for digestion and assimilation, it curbs hunger, helps build muscle, is delicious ... I think I'll include protein in my day!

Fat

Don't be hatin' here! While this macro doesn't get spread around too well in the media (yes that was a butter joke, did I get any courtesy chuckles?), it has some major roles in helping your body, mind, and taste buds. Avocado, walnuts, olive oil- these are some examples with which you are probably familiar.

One day you hear fat is carcinogenic, the next day fats from fish can stop Alzheimer's in its tracks, so what's the real deal? The truth is that we NEED fat! When you look at its necessity for our hormone production and brain health, this macro has a starring role in our daily lives.

So, if it's good for you, then more is better, right? Especially if it's organic and from the "good fat" kind, I can have as much as I want and the gains will keep on coming, right? NO! Well, you'll get gains, but not the kind you're looking for, more so on the waistline. Too much fat is just that: too much fat! Excess intake will be stored as bodyfat, whether it's organic coconut oil or lard. Essential fatty acids, yes, they are essential! Let's not lose sight of this concept, however: too much is too much! Just because it has benefits, it's still a fat. The keyword here is **moderation**. Say it with me, now!

Putting it all together, we have a mix of the 3 macros in almost every meal (and individual food, for that matter) that we eat. That is the beauty of flexible dieting: focus on the macros, and you can make your meals how you like them! I would like to take a moment and define what this does NOT mean: eating garbage all day because "it fit my macros." A similar moniker to flexible dieting is IIFYM: If It Fits Your Macros, NOT If It Fits Your Mouth!

Flexible is good because it allows you to enjoy some indulgences, within moderation, and still stay on track with your nutrition, health, and wellness goals. Is eating on a rigid, "all clean" and restrictive diet good for your overall wellness? Well, let me ask you this: have you tried doing that? If you have, I bet you felt like you were going insane, even starving yourself! Most likely it was because in effect, you were.

Where's the middle ground, then? Taking the flexible dieting approach with moderation and realizing that eating PopTarts® for all meals of the day is not a healthy approach, I recommend using the **80/20 rule of thumb**: 80% of your intake being from wholesome, nutrient-dense foods (sweet potato, fish, veggies) and 20% being those often-labeled "forbidden foods." Have you ever been to a wedding? Had wedding cake? Well, if you were "all clean" you're telling me that if you're getting married you won't "cheat" and enjoy your own wedding cake? That you paid for? Are you getting that this sounds a little ridiculous? How about more practical applications: socializing with friends, birthday parties, work functions, eating out with your family? There IS a solution, and that, my friends, is flexible dieting![1]

Well what ratio of each macro should I eat?

Here lies the beauty of flexible dieting: it depends on YOU! Your body type, eating preferences, metabolism, eating history, goals... the list goes on! That is where we come in at The Fit Pharmacist: we work with you as an individual to customize your macro ranges! No cookie cutter, copy-paste programs here- we recognize that every person is vastly different from one another (just look at the above variables) so we take the time to do an extensive intake regarding these. We then work with you, at your own pace, to help you develop the skills, know-how and experience to become your own best nutritionist. We believe in self-empowerment rather than relying on an expensive shake, skinny wrap, or fad diet.

Working from science-based research, and being in business for over 25 years with a RD, MD, PharmD, PhD in psychology, and exercise physiologist on staff, we collectively come together to bring you the best science and support to turn your wellness wishes into reality! To learn more, check out www.thefitpharmacist.com

*Disclaimer: this is for informational purposes only. While TheFitPharmacist has a registered dietician on staff, laws do not allow the "prescribing" or consultations of diets or eating strategies by anyone other than a registered dietician (RD). Please consult your state laws to learn more.

VI. ℞: Stay Up-to-Date and Validate Your Resources

Nutrition Know-How: Be Aware of What Information to Avoid

Nutrition: something that every human being needs as a part of their daily life for optimal health, and something that almost every human strives to improve. So, the demand for sound knowledge is there, but when it comes to supply, it unfortunately is lacking when it comes to quality. How many times this month alone have you seen a headline related to nutrition? How about this week? Today, even? It seems that one day a certain food is touted as a cure-all, and the next it is carcinogenic- *which facts are right? Which facts are wrong? Are they even "facts" at all to begin with?!*

The media is in business to grow their business, and as consumer's attention/eyeballs are the common real estate up for grabs, flashy headlines, outlandish claims, and facts that go completely against conventional wisdom are big ticket options. All this really does is add to the never-ending pool of misinformation, causation inappropriately derived from correlation, and even MORE confusion about answering the simple question of "What should I eat". In our days where everyone is a "nutritionist", "foodie expert", and "health coach", it can be hard to discern what is real and backed by actual science and what was regurgitated from Suzy Q's Twitter feed.

I'm here to set the record straight about how YOU can easily identify what information is real, what is make believe, and things to look for when evaluating the latest nutrition news. Take it as a grain of salt (oh the puns never stop), but regardless of the topic or claim, these facets of fact finding will hold true so that you can be empowered with the real deal and not fake news.

Key Questions to Ask When Evaluating Nutrition News:
1.   Who's who?
Social media can create the illusion that the person posting the infomeme or hashtag actually discovered the groundbreaking knowledge nugget that will change how humans eat food forever. #notsofast

Before you take what you read as gospel, you must first determine the validity of the source: is the person making the claim a qualified professional in the field of interest? If the information was online, who manages the website and where does the content come from? Are the names of the article's authors clearly listed and cited with their credentials? Is the information posted/published reviewed for accuracy or was it just up as a guest blog piece from the owner's sister-in-law?

2.   We're not in Kansas no mo'! Where?
Have you ever heard the catch phrase *"consider the source"*? How about "its cliché because it's true"? Do you see what I did there?! When it comes to online information, it is indeed the go-to source for the majority of Americans, as an estimated 2 out of 3 adults use it to research health information or learn it from- believe it or not- online chat groups.[1] As we all (I hope) know, rather unfortunately, the online world is riddled with incorrect data, misleading claims, and downright inaccurate conclusions inappropriately drawn from published studies.[3] Remember how not too long ago we said everyone nowadays is a "nutritionist" etc.? Well, now

everyone is an author, too! Publishing anything can be done by anyone, anywhere- fun fact to consider. I promise, though- I'm legit, fellow readers!

3.   A Wrinkle In Time- When?

Just like fashion, nutrition data can go out of date. I know, I know- Twinkies® still aren't the cure all, but you never know! When you are reading an article on nutrition, it is always a good idea to consider *when* that data was published. Is it the most current? If not, it's possible that there are new findings, as study after study is conducted relentlessly on the multifaceted era of nutrition. It is an evolving science, and with that, you want to ensure you are getting the most current information- based on quality information, of course. Checking to see when the article or website was last updated is a good idea to ensure it is on the up-and-up so that you can be, too.

4.   Why? Why Not? Why else?

While there are plenty of good-intentioned people out there striving to provide you with the best information without asking for anything in return, information-based marketing has become extremely popular for businesses worldwide. That is, we give you information that ties directly to our product explaining the benefits and how great it is, then we ask for the sale. It's not wrong and I'm not chastising it, but you need to be aware of WHY that information is being presented to you. Ask yourself if the source of your information is there for the sole purpose of education, or is it a website looking to sell you a product? While there are companies that provide quality information that is legitimately tied to their product or service for sale, unfortunately there are far more that do not and offer a one-sided glimpse of a study's results that leave you feeling like you cannot LIVE without buying their offer! If you find by asking *"what's the why"* that the main motivation is money, proceed with caution that the information presented to you may not be telling you the whole story- just the side the leads to the sale.

5. "YeaaYaaaaa… Oooookkkkk… WHAT?!?" (ode to Lil' John)

If the "fact" that grabbed your attention seems to be complete opposite of what has been known for a while, proceed with caution. That's not to say that it's wrong per se, but remember: eyeballs are in high competition for rankings and clicks. Ask yourself what the overall message in the headline/article is and if it's backed up by sources outside of itself (i.e., not an outlier being reported as a study's overall outcome). If it is reliable, often times you will find its claims backed up by having links to other sources touting the same conclusions. Now, just having links does NOT mean it's true, but see where they lead, and assess that site's validity using the same questions we are going through now. Hyperlinking is as free as breathing air is for you and me- there are no stipulations, so again, proceed with caution!

General Warnings to Watch For
Email is effective for many helpful reasons- it saves time, is immediate, and can be a great route of communication. It's also effective at spreading "scarelore"- false facts that aim to grab your attention, usually for the purpose of either selling something or someone looking to become famous. Effective, not helpful- here's what to watch for:
- It was forwarded from a long chain of previous senders
- You don't know the original source

- The original source isn't stated, cited or has any supportive credentials
- "Forward this if you don't want bad luck... only to those you care about..." you get the idea
- The information is astonishing or shocking compared to what you know from legitimate informants
- There! ARE! A TONNN!!! Of e!x!c!l!a!m!a!t!i!o!n! POINTS!!! Or verbiage that aims to evoke heightened senses of awareness or emotion
- References are lacking or seem questionable if provided
- The information has already been discredited- check the following websites to weed out the whacky: www.quackwatch.org, www.snoops.com, www.urbanlegends.com

With Billions of Websites, Which One Is Worthy?!

While yes, there are many websites that deliver quality information that is accurate, that is followed by a "OH MY YES" when it comes to the number of inaccurate websites offering information lacking validity. Using the above questions will help you to identify fact from fiction in the world of nutrition as you encounter fact after fact, from apples to zucchini. A safe bet as a reputable resource is the US National Library of Medicine's PubMed, delivering FREE access to over 23 million abstracts from research papers actually published in legitimate journals worldwide. You can find it online at www.pubmed.gov along with tutorials that will assist you if you're a first-timer here on how to best access the information in the database. Another option is to simply go to the site and Google-fy it, through simply typing in what you're looking for in the "Search for" box at the top, click "Go", and sift your results. Both are viable options to find accurate information for whatever your heart- or stomach- desires.

Fake News Is New News

Again, we go back to the why mentioned earlier and the competition for eyeballs in the media. Which would you rather watch:

"Studies show eating an apple a day is linked to improved overall health"

Or

"Pink slime infests the meat supply of the United States"

Often times there IS some truth in what the media delivers, however it is also often out of context, skewed, and reported before the actual data is delivered in a whole-context complete picture of what the research actually found and what conclusions can be drawn, rather than making a causation out of a correlation.

When the headline begins with "new study finds…" it often is the correlative findings from ONE study in a SPECIFIC circumstance, population or niche that has not yet been replicated by other researchers. This makes the headline both current and controversial, something as modern humans we innately thrive on when it comes to our attention.

Tell me how many times this week alone you've seen a "new finding" that completely contradicts the verified facts that have held true for the last 20+ years- pretty confusing, isn't it? Contradictions are what we are primed to gravitate toward, and the media uses this to shift our eyeballs their way. Yes, ONE single study may have found something different- but the thing we must *always* remember is **context**. The facts as we know them and are taught do not come from one single study, but from multiple studies from a diversity of researchers and settings that have been successfully replicated to verify the findings time and time again. Dr. Whitney and Dr. Rolfe say it best in the following excerpt:

"A single study contributes to the big picture, but when viewed alone, it can easily distort the image. To be meaningful the conclusions of any study must be presented cautiously within the context of other research findings."

Consider the Source- Continued

We had mentioned credentials being important when discerning advice or information as accurate- again, context is key. Just because someone is a "doctor" does NOT mean they know everything about everything! "Doctor" of what? Google? What makes someone a nutrition expert, anyway?

Often times when we hear the word "doctor" we are conditioned to associate it with "physician", who are excellent resources for many health-related matters. When it comes to nutrition guidance, you must consider if they are specialized in that arena of health or if that is their area of expertise- there are a lot of disease states, medications, procedures and policies to know! One thing to note regarding this profession is that across all medical schools in the United States:

- **Less than 1/3** require their medical students to take a separate nutrition course
- **Less than 1/2** require them to take the required 25 hours minimum of nutrition instruction that is recommended by the National Academy of Sciences

Compare these students with those in a registered dietician program who are enrolled in a nutrition course that provides 45 hours of instruction, on average, and who are you going to ask about apples or oranges?

Let's not throw the baby out with the bath water just yet! The Academy of Nutrition and Dietetics emphasizes that standardized nutrition education should be integrated into the curriculum of schools across all healthcare professions who directly provide care to patients. Once nutrition knowledge as it relates to disease prevention is paired with their area of expertise, everyone will be better equipped to live healthier lives with empowerment through this information.

With that being said, if you are a fellow healthcare practitioner (and by reading this book I suspect you are), you're probably thinking *"We barely had enough time to fit in all of the information specific to my field as it was! How can we expect to add even one lecture more let alone nutrition as a whole?!"* This is the beauty of interprofessional communication, referring when necessary, and knowing where your passions do and do not reside. Time and experience are of the essence, and if developing the skills required to successfully create diet plans/provide related counseling to patients is not in the picture, a qualified nutrition expert such as a Registered Dietitian (RD) would be a great professional to have in your network!

A RD is recognized by the Academy of Nutrition and Dietetics (AND) to "have the educational background necessary to deliver reliable nutrition advice and care."[4] In order to become a registered dietitian, one must first earn an undergraduate degree consisting of ~60 credit hours based in nutrition, food science, or related areas, then complete a year-long clinical internship, pass a national examination administered by the AND, then stay up-to-date with their experience and registration through accredited continuing education endeavors (e.g. courses, research, seminars).

As you have read, earning the title "registered dietitian" is no small feat! That is why the term 'dietitian' is *legally protected* in the majority of states in America. In addition, some require a state registration, or **license to practice**: "permission under state or federal law, granted on meeting specified criteria, to use a certain title (i.e. dietitian) and offer certain services."[5] With the point of this section being how to identify real vs fake nutrition information, entire states in our country have taken it upon themselves to distinguish the sources of nutrition information – the people themselves offering and performing related specified duties- through legal certification! States can literally identify professionals who are credentialed, legitimate, and proven to have the appropriate skills and knowledge necessary to make responsible suggestions regarding nutrition to those seeking advice to improve their own health. This is not the ONLY credentials one may obtain to be identified as well-versed in nutrition- there is also certified nutritionist, certified nutritional consultant, or certified nutrition therapist- which sound official, but do not warrant as much legal rights as that of a registered dietitian. Each of these three terms simply label an individual as someone who has been declared authority as a nutrition professional.

Just as a pharmacist has pharmacy technicians, a dietitian has a dietitian technician, registered (DTR) who functions to assist the RD in their roles and responsibilities. Only after a dietitian technician has worked under a RD and passed a national examination does s/he earn the ", *registered*" after their title, much like a *certified* pharmacy technician would gain the extra credentials from "pharmacy technician".

We have defined the legitimate sources of information from a credentialed standpoint- that is, for the individual touting nutrition advice. When it comes to *groups* of people who are deemed credible sources of information, there are fortunately many to choose from! Government agencies, volunteer associations, consumer groups, and professional organizations deliver accurate data related to diet that can be helpful for consumers.

I leave you with these questions to consider as you encounter more and more information in your daily pursuit of better understanding nutrition, health and wellness – some food for thought:

If something sounds counterintuitive, radical or is a big claim, what thought process of analysis will you use to determine if it's worth considering as valid?

TABLE H1-1 Credible Sources of Nutrition Information

Government agencies, volunteer associations, consumer groups, and professional organizations provide consumers with reliable health and nutrition information. Credible sources of nutrition information include:

- Nutrition and food science departments at a university or community college
- Local agencies such as the health department or County Cooperative Extension Service
- Government health agencies such as:
  - Department of Agriculture (USDA)   www.usda.gov
  - Department of Health and Human   www.os.dhhs.gov
    Services (DHHS)
  - Food and Drug Administration (FDA)   www.fda.gov
  - Health Canada   www.hc-sc.gc.ca/nutrition
- Volunteer health agencies such as:
  - American Cancer Society   www.cancer.org
  - American Diabetes Association   www.diabetes.org
  - American Heart Association   www.americanheart.org

- Reputable consumer groups such as:
  - American Council on Science and Health   www.acsh.org
  - Federal Citizen Information Center   www.pueblo.gsa.gov
  - International Food Information Council   www.ific.org
- Professional health organizations such as:
  - American Dietetic Association   www.eatright.org
  - American Medical Association   www.ama-assn.org
  - Dietitians of Canada   www.dietitians.ca
- Journals such as:
  - *American Journal of Clinical Nutrition*   www.ajcn.org
  - *Journal of the American Dietetic Association*   www.adajournal.org
  - *New England Journal of Medicine*   www.nejm.org
  - *Nutrition Reviews*   www.ilsi.org

Table H1-1: Credible Sources of Nutrition Information. Adapted from "Understanding Nutrition" by E Whitney and S. R. Rolfes, 2016, p. 33. Copyright 2016 by Cengage Learning

VII. ℞: Overcome Barriers Keeping You from Becoming Physically Fit

Myths and Misconceptions Keeping You From Physical Fitness

"I'm so busy- I don't have TIME to workout!"

If this is you, I HAVE THE SOLUTION!! As a lifetime drug-free competitive bodybuilder of 12 years, who also works full-time as a pharmacist, I have heard this before, but did NOT let "lack of time" stop me from staying on track with my physical fitness. Any yes, YOU can fit it in, too! My niche is helping people who default to "I just don't have enough time" realize that yes, yes they do- by using SimpleSolutions - health hacks and strategies that allow you to MAXIMIZE your time through optimization and helpful tips and tricks that are both *practical* and *actually work*!

I teamed up with the most passionate professional I know when it comes to physical fitness- along with the experience and credentials to back up his input! He is THE expert- so much so, that I have personally worked with him as my strength and programming coach for over 4 years. The man I speak of is coach Luke E. Propst, the training director of The Diet Doc, LLC and owner of Predator Strength Training. A little about this master of muscle:

Luke Propst, MS, CSCS was bit by the Iron Bug at 15 and has spent the last 25 years under a heavy barbell. In the course of pursuing his master's degree in exercise physiology and more training certifications than he can remember he has worked with everything from Division 1 college athletes, rehab and performance settings, youth athletes, and bodybuilders, powerlifters, endurance athletes and weekend warriors. He is always looking to learn more practical information to help his clients reach their goals safely, efficiently, and with a lifelong love of learning and fitness. You can reach him directly at luke@thedietdoc.com

Together, we identified the most common myths, misconceptions, and *PERCEIEVED* barriers that seem to get in the way of making your workouts happen. I present to you now the most commonly perceived barriers I hear from healthcare professionals who want to fit in fitness, but can't seem to find the time! Let's dive right in:

1. **You have to workout for 1 to 2 hours 5 days per week to get any noticeable results.**

With a belief like that, you're right: WHO has time for that, ESPECIALLY if you work in healthcare?! So if the above isn't true, *how long does your workout have to be in order for it to be effective?*

Let's set the record straight with some fact-based knowledge bombs:

The "best" duration for a workout is the one that an individual can consistently implement and execute on a consistent basis. In order to make that happen, it's best to adapt to a timeframe that is realistic for your specific lifestyle, and be able to make on-the-fly adjustments to that baseline structure in order to get in a safe and efficient workout with the time that you have in that moment in order to properly execute your exercises. So to start, it's best to have the structure of a good workout routine from a qualified professional catered to YOUR specific goals and abilities as an individual, *paired* with the flexibility to make changes as needed depending on your day, biofeedback, or changes in goals as time goes on.

2. **You have to warmup for 20 minutes before your workout AND cool-down for 20 minutes after, and that is time I do not have let alone for the workout itself!**

Rules are meant to be broken- especially if they're not based on research, which the above time frames are absolutely not! That, then, leads to some great questions:

How long should my warm up and cool down be? WHY do I even have to do either? Can I skip one or both to save time without adding risk?

The Warm-Up:
Warming up properly does NOT mean just jumping on the treadmill; it's going through a movement that simulates the work that you are about to do. This way, if there are any issues/tight muscles that need addressed prior to the workout, they can be appropriately handled through a more specific warm up routine. It's kind of like diagnostics- looks at that healthcare relevance!

So what's best to do is to warm up specific to the movement you're about to perform in your workout. For example, if you're going to be doing upper body work, you don't necessarily need to focus all of your time on warming up your calves. Focus on the muscles you're about to use, in a movement pattern that 'primes' them to be ready to go. A good warm-up needs to focus on increasing blood flow to the soon-to-be-working muscles. [6]

The Cool Down:

Yes, it's necessary for optimal recovery from your workout, but it does NOT have to be excessive. How long, you may ask? 5 minutes is plenty.

WHY even do it? Well, the purpose of cooling down after your workout is that you're trying to redirect the blood that was shuttled to your working muscles (arms, legs, etc.) back to your core. You know, where all of your organs are at- priorities for the goods have now shifted, you fitness fanatic!

WHAT to do? It's extremely beneficial to practice diaphragmatic breathing while lying on the floor so you can bring yourself back to center, and into a calm state following your intense workout (oh yes, I am betting it was intense- of course it was, you rockstar).

3. Stretching is such a waste- I'm NOT trying to be a gymnast or "bend it like Beckham"!

Whoa there, Gumby- let's take a look at this real quick! Specifically, some common questions that come up when it comes to stretching are:

Is stretching really necessary? WHAT do I even do, and WHEN do I do it (before/after the workout)?

WHAT to do? Some gentle, static stretching is a great way to redistribute blood flow back to the center of your body (as we discussed the why in the cool down section above). With that being said, we come to an important aspect of stretching: the *WHEN*.

Word of Caution: You do NOT want to do static stretching BEFORE your work out- this will reduce work output (unless you are in a dangerous position, and need to address mobility restrictions). Again, the components of an efficient workout are a moving target with the *structure* of principles, implemented through *flexibility* depending on the individual and the specific situation.[7]

4. There are SO many workout protocols/plans out there. Which one is "best"?

Why would you put all of your time, effort and energy if it wasn't the Rolls Royce® plan, am I right?! Well, not quite- the beauty of "best" is in the eye- er, that is the *muscles* and *respiratory system*- of the beholder. Let Luke explain:

What is the best program? <u>Answer</u>: the one you're not on.

In general, every workout program is going to have strengths and weaknesses. When you then apply it to the individual, it becomes dependent on *their* goals, *their* enjoyment of the routine, and their ability to *consistently* implement said program.

When we then take a program or standard routine and aim to make it optimal or "the best", there must be some degree of individualization to the person, and the workout they have. It does NOT have to be black and white- "do it this way or it won't work/don't waste your time if you can't XYZ."

What we're saying is this: if fitting in a workout is the most preventative factor for you, there is a SimpleSolution! You can break it up into sections. For example, if you do not have 40 minutes for a workout, you can do 20 minutes in the morning, and 20 minutes in the evening, and *still* get the same benefits! How about that for problem solving?

The main principle to keep in mind is this: when setting up a program, it's NOT a question of what is the best *physiologically*- but really, what is the best in terms of whether the individual will actually do it and implement it on a _consistent_ basis.

The other secret ingredient is hard work- that is, really _working_ your work out! If you work hard at a sub-par program, you are going to do better than if you half-ass an elite, "perfect" program hands down- even if on paper it's "the best possible program that could ever be created for you".

Succinctly put: **consistent effort beats wishful thinking**.

Getting the work done in _your_ time, _over_ time, is what will lead to results!

5. When it comes to lifting weights, use high reps for 'toning', and low reps for strength and size.

Dude no! This _does_ present some phenomenal questions when it comes to the exercises in your workout routine: _what rep ranges (number of repetitions performed) are best for getting "toned"?_

You can build muscle BOTH with low-weight/high-reps OR heavy-weight/low-reps. The difference in your results will ultimately depend on your overall volume. If you are using very heavy weights to build muscle as your goal, that will take a very long time to accomplish- you will have to rest longer in between sets in order to get the equivalent volume as opposed to using a lighter weight ('volume' meaning number of overall repetitions for a given exercise).

TONING: There is no "toning" or ways that will magically get you a certain way. Muscles adapt, and they will respond to the stimulus and volume that you give them! The human body is an amazing organism- I know, I know, you know that, you healthcare professional- but it warrants being pointed out regardless!

With that being said, we can tie that to the question at hand relating to your workout: you can get the SAME results with *either* light OR heavy weights- the difference comes down to length of time for each, and whether you will enjoy one process over the other, because THAT will lead to compliance and long-term success.
8

Here's the good news: it doesn't have to be all black and white! You are not tied down to one or the other, heavy or light. It's actually best to have a mix of both- again, depending on the individual, their goals, and being realistic with the time they have to consistently adhere to their program.

WHICH IS BEST THO?
It's very beneficial to incorporate hi-repetition movement ranges into your routine. If there is "the best" it would be to add this in some fashion to your program. But again, the main point is that it's NOT a black-and-white, this-is-right /that-is-wrong approach. Say it with me now: *structured flexibility*.

6. **If I am a woman and then lift weights, I will turn into a man.**

One of THE most common myths in the fitness world: "Women shouldn't lift weights if they don't want to become manly."

This is DEFINITELY one we will address head-on, because weight lifting has SO many benefits- not only for your health, but to most efficiently forge the physique you are working so hard to achieve!

If that's not true, then why are some women who lift weights so muscular? I do NOT want to look like a man and lose my feminine figure!

Fear of weightlifting causing too much muscle growth: it doesn't just "accidentally happen"- women have different hormonal profiles than men, which lead to different rates and capacities for muscle growth. Now, *among* women, some DO have an easier time gaining muscle (again, varying hormone levels). So, if you find that with weightlifting you are gaining more muscle than you are comfortable with, the SimpleSolution would be to tone back your volume and intensity. That's it, that simple! You are NOT going to be "stuck that way forever"- it is not a trap that you can "fall into". Weight lifting affords SO many health benefits that it would be a shame for you not to use this tool to yield rapid results on your quest for efficiently forging your physique!

7. When it comes to cardio or weights, just pick one- they both get you fit, and time is limited!

Tick-tock goes the clock, and bye-bye go the options if you approach fitness with a limited scope of potential using an "either/or" lens of possibility. So then you ask:

Do I HAVE to do cardio AND weights?

CARDIO- that is, *cardiovascular exercise*, has MANY health benefits. Now, that does not mean you have to live on a treadmill or use any equipment confining you to a gym. Walking your dog, mowing the grass, doing yardwork or being immersed in nature where you get your heart rate increased for a moderately prolonged period of time are all potential options for you to pick from that will allow you to get cardiovascular benefits.

Cardio does not have to be in the same session as weight lifting. For example, if you only have 30 minutes, it does not have to be evenly divided into 15 minutes for weight lifting, 15 minutes for cardio. Stick with the weights for 30 minutes, then you can find many other creative ways to get in movement that can be counted as cardio at other times of the day. Look at that: structured flexibility yet again!

Cardio does have many health benefits- however, when it comes to changing your physique as your main goal, it is not a requirement. You CAN get phenomenal results through nutrition and weight training alone. You do not have to live on a treadmill or pump your legs like a gazelle on the elliptical (you know EXACTLY what I'm talking about here)! There are many other creative and enjoyable ways to fit cardio into your lifestyle- it's all about that flexibility.

Summing up everything that we just broke down in the specifics of physical activity, fitting in physical fitness for the pharmacist comes down to this simple fact:

What time you have- the time you can carve out, create and dedicate to working out- is what will make the difference long-term- even if it's less time than you think is needed for 'real results'. It's not black-and-white, whereas if you can't work out for three hours it's not going to yield any results. Consistently committing to what you CAN do is what will make all the difference! Realistically decide how much time you do you have, carve that out and set it aside, and create a plan so that you can stick to it with that structure in place.

Go forth and be fit, my friends.

Now that we have debunked the mainstream misconception, we can now get into SimpleSolutions for HOW to actually fit in physical fitness to the demanding lifestyle of a Fit Pharmacist-to-be!

VIII. ℞: Fit In Physical Fitness to Your Routine

How to Fit in Fitness as A Pharmacist

With all of the 30 different tasks we are expected to do all at once as pharmacists, HOW can we even think of adding one more task to our plate- let alone something that requires 30-60 minutes of our time 3-5 days per week?!? Insanity? Unrealistic? Impossible? So, one may think. But as a pharmacist who has worked full-time in the community setting for close to a decade, competing in 4 bodybuilding competitions, I have found some super simple tricks that have enabled myself- and those I work with as a nutrition consultant and personal trainer- to master their management in making fitness a consistent part of their personal wellness script for success!

The key: **consistency**. But HOW DO YOU FIND THE TIME? It's not about living in the gym- in fact, studies repeatedly show that 86% of Americans have NO interest in ever going to a gym at all! That's right: *86%!* It's not a black and white solution: the gym is one option available, but it's not a "you have to do it or else"- it's about finding some physical activity that you *enjoy*, because if you like doing it, you'll likely *keep* doing it! Repetition is the mother of skill, so we want to make sure you continually get all of your reps in!

Here are some SimpleSolutions you can fit in to your daily routine that will best align you to fit fitness into your life as a pharmacist:

1.   **The shortest distance between 2 points is a straight line**
That is, if you're trying to get in a workout after your shift at ClubPharmacy, go STRAIGHT to your workout! Whether it's to the gym, outside for a walk, or lacing up those Silver Sneakers for some laps at the mall, **one of the most effective ways to ensuring that**

happens is to go straight from work to your workout. That means packing your workout clothes and gear to take with you to work! You can either change at the pharmacy at the end of your shift or have your gym bag packed in your car so you have everything you'll need for a great workout!

But I'll just stop at home really quick after work...
Have you ever tried that, and sat down to just tie your shoes, and then the reasons for staying put start to flood your mind? For most, just sitting ONE TIME means "game over" for the workout plans- stay in the game, stay on your way to make it happen!

2.   Proper Preparation Prevents Poor Performance
You can't successfully follow through with the first tip if you don't pack your gym back with all of the essentials to make the workout even happen! What do I mean? Well, the *exact* equipment will vary from person to person, but for 99% of us, use the following gym bag checklist to ensure you are packed for peak performance:

- Workout clothes: shorts, shirt, jacket/sweats if cold
- Water bottle
- Headphones
- Music with a great beat
- Post workout snack/protein
- Digital watch/stopwatch
- Jump rope
- Lifting gloves/wrist wraps/straps if desired
- Shaker cup/mixing bottle
- Small towel – you DO plan on sweating it out, yes?!

3.   If it's important to you, you'll make it happen; if not, you'll make an excuse
Here is one fun fact: we all have the same amount of willpower! That is, it's a limited resource that weans off as the day goes on (I'm

sure you know this already from experience! Err, so your neighbor said?). With that being said, if you know that you'll be using up a lot before the end of the day, and you just can't find it in you to get a workout in after work, **prioritize hitting your workout first thing in the morning.** This is a great way to get your blood flowing, set you up for success for the rest of the day, and you will feel super accomplished knowing that your workout is already in the books before the sun has finished rising! Nothing can stop you now!

4. No coffee, no workee-out-ee

Off all of the hundreds and thousands of shimmery, fancy pre-workout supplements on the market today, one beats them all and is backed by repeatedly proven scientific studies touting its effectiveness: **caffeine!** Of course, if you have certain medical conditions or are taking certain medications, you should avoid this and always consult your physician before starting ANY supplement of any kind (but you know this, fellow pharmacist!), but devoid of contraindications, this will add some serious focus, fat burning and energy to your workout to enable you to reap the max benefits from your commitment to excellence. It's not a "must", but it sure does fuel the fire for fitness!

5. Blame Someone Else

That's right, s/he did it- I know you are innocent! *"Huh?"*

What I mean is that studies have shown over and over again that of the people who have successfully developed the habit of working out consistently have reported having an accountability/workout partner. Decades of research later still names this one trait as one of the most common success habits of those who follow through on their workout plans. This keeps people on track with physical fitness programs for many reasons, but **psychology** is the strong driving force here: we all have days (yes, me too!) when we just do NOT feel like working out- but if our spouse/neighbor/friend is counting on us to show up, we will grin and bear it to keep our word to our workout partner. Buddy up, giddy up, and go! BONUS: you social butterfly, you!

6.   Be Like Chronos and Optimize Your Time

Ok, Ok, Greek mythology is still alive here with that reference! But if you are trying to get in a really solid, complete workout and incorporate weight lifting, cardio, and vary your intensity, but find that doing all of those things separately is just not realistic with your time, say hello to combination magic! There are several workout regimens, gyms, and clubs that combine these and more into one 30- or 60-minute workout for maximum efficiency. OrangeTheoryFitness and CrossFit are just two examples, but this is yet another option you can use to make the magic happen and fit it into your schedule!

BONUS: if you decide to join one of these clubs, get there early to meet those in your class, and BOOM you just added in tip #5 and gained an accountability partner (or two or more). Look at you combining steps- super efficient at becoming efficient! Well done, FitPharmFam!

7.   Go on: You DESERVE IT!

Now, I KNOW this an ironic statement as we're talking about fitness and this line is usually what your friends say to you when you're out for ice cream and YOU are on a diet and THEY are NOT, but really look at what that says. YOU DESERVE IT! The most important investment you will EVER make is in yourself, and you can't perform optimally, regardless of what your "performance" is if your body is not healthy. You only get one body in this life: it is a tool to help others, to carry out your life's work, and your temple to serve- treat it well! Reading this book, I think it is safe to assume that you work in pharmacy or healthcare and therefore seek to serve others. Have you ever heard the phrase, *"You cannot pour from an empty cup"*? That means you gotta take care of YOU, boo! You make serving others a priority, but don't neglect taking care of yourself.

If you DO seek to prioritize your health and wellness, this will only better align you and your body to perform at its 100% potential, which will in turn allow you to provide the very best care possible to those you serve and interact with in your daily life. This belief is the core of what it means to be a FitPharmacist, and the whole reason I created TheFitPharmacist movement! To help each other through our obstacles we face as pharmacists, to inspire each other and support each other in reaching our own optimal health as healthcare professionals so that we can better optimize the health of those we serve. YOU can do this too- *and* inspire those you work with and serve to reach their highest level of health!

IX. Final ℞: Dispense Your Greatness QDay (refills: PRN)

How to Implement the Above, Stay Consistent With Your Rx for Health, and Fill Your Full Potential

Hey, community pharmacists- we are THE masters at counting by 5's, so what better way to keep simple with consistency than by focusing on 5 SimpleSolutions that collectively will script you an IRONCLAD method to ALWAYS follow through on your goals! BONUS: this formula can go beyond your health- you will find that it can be successfully applied to your business, personal development, relationships and beyond. No reconstitution required.

You are probably reading this book and have gotten this far because you are HUNGRY for health, for mastering your mindset and feeling your absolute best! That is a goal, and all too often "goal" leads to "resolution" which can be postponed until New Years. ALERT! You do NOT have to wait until January 1 to set out on your goal- in fact, you would not want to anyway: *80% of people who start a New Year's resolution quit by February 15!*

Here are 5 Key Elements- SimpleSolutions- that when combined and put into action, will **GUARANTEE** that you WILL follow through with your goal, whatever it may be, straight through to success:

1.   Write YOUR Rx
That's right: script out what you WANT! Set your target, and then re-commit to your target and purpose every single day. Physically write out these 2 things- the what and the why-

on a habitual daily basis. In order to help you get really clear on these, consider these questions to ask yourself:

WHY are you doing what you're doing?

WHAT will your ideal outcome to be?

Imagine you reached your goal- how will you feel once that is accomplished?

2.   Control Your Half Life.

Hold it together for short periods of time. 24 hours. Literally, this simple mindset shift will make SUCH a difference for you in sticking to your goals! Consider 2 options, A and B:

A: I only have to stick to my workout plan and nutrition goals for 24 hours

B: I have to hit ALL of my workouts for 2 years, and not stray from my nutrition plan for 2 whole years.

Which one sounded simple- like a super easy challenge that you WANT to accomplish for the sake of accomplishment?

Which one gave you literal disgust, anxiety, and maybe even a feeling of restricted freedom?

If you only focus on holding it together for short periods of time- asking yourself "what is my job for this one hour...for this work shift... for this day until I go to bed tonight" doesn't that seem so much more simple? So much less daunting? So much more inviting of success? Once you follow through on that, guess what: you've just created **momentum**, which will carry over into tomorrow so that you can hold it together for *another* short period of time. Each success will fuel the next, and before you know it, you'll have success so powerful others will take notice! Just hang in there until you get to the next round.

Now, even if you are focused on holding it together for short periods of time, thoughts and temptations will probably sneak into the equation. I'm sure you are really good at convincing yourself to do things, maybe even things that don't always align with your main goal (for example, I DESERVE this extra pint of ice cream for the workout I did- in addition to the half cake I just ate). SO, it would be a good idea to…

3.   Formulate accountability

Have someone hold you accountable – specifically, someone other than yourself! If you have a coach, someone you respect, or a loved one, it will be a lot harder to cave in to actions not in line with your end goal vs having that convincing conversation with yourself when you may be tired, be low on "willpower" or had to pull a double shift without expecting it (that NEVER happens in healthcare of course)- this will pay dividends when it comes to consistency over the long term in sticking to your goals. And as we know, consistency is the magic bullet for success!

You can simplify this even further and not even ask to do it! You don't need to ask their permission: just having that person around you that inspires you or that you look up to could be all that it takes for you, just to be around the right people! Their actions will keep you accountable because they are setting examples of doing more, inspiring you to do the same. Free advice right here for free accountability- you can find it wherever you need it!

4.   Set Your Future Fill Date

That is, have something to look forward to in the future! Keep yourself focused on the future towards progress by planning a scheduled event. Tie the event to achieving your goal to add another layer of accountability to yourself so that you follow through. Signing up for a marathon, fitness competition, or scheduling a sporting event are just some examples for how you can tie your fitness goal and progress to something you look forward to- just keep it specific to YOU!

5.   **Focus on Your Rx**

Never take your eye off the ball- you took time and energy to take the actions needed to create momentum, implement the habits in your daily life that led you to progress toward your goal. Just because you met your goal, that does NOT mean it is time to quit or rest on your laurels! Success can be dangerous if it leads to too much comfort- **those who succeed party, those who fail ponder**. Now, I'm not saying not to take notice of all of the amazing progress and success you've earned! Why stop there? What's next: keep that goal weight/performance endurance? Run faster? Get more creative with your cooking skills? Try a new area of fitness? Write a book on health and wellness :D ? **Your potential is only limited by the limits you place on yourself!**

Resources:

With that being said, I can certainly understand and appreciate when we ARE thinking of "what's next?" and get stuck on which direction to go next. Sometimes, we just need some ideas or inspiration that spark us into that "AHA, that's it!" moment that propels us forward to the next first step. Here are some of those resources that may be of service to you as you continue your journey toward excellence beyond what you may have ever thought possible:

The Diet Doc:
>   www.thedietdoc.com

The Fit Pharmacist
>   www.thefitpharmacist.com

The Diet Doc Life Mastery Podcast
>   On all audio platforms!

The Fit Pharmacist Healthcare Podcast
>   On all audio platforms!

Bulk Cooking:
https://thefitpharmacist.com/how-to-meal-prep-for-work

YouTube Channels for Mindset Mastery:
>   The Diet Doc Permanent Weight Loss
>   The Fit Pharmacist

Identify Discredited Nutrition Information:
>   www.quackwatch.org
>   www.snoops.com
>   www.urbanlegends.com

Legitimate Nutrition Article References:
>   www.pubmed.gov

References:

1. Klemczewski J, Propst K. 50 Days to Your Best Life! Evansville: Word Spank, 2014. Print.

2. R. A. Cohen and P. F. Adams, Use of the Internet for health information: United States, 2009, *NCHS Data Brief*, July 2011.

3. Practice paper of the Academy of Nutrition and Dietetics abstract: Communicating accurate food and nutrition information, *Journal of the Academy of Nutrition and Dietetics* 112 (2012): 759.

4. Position of the Academy of Nutrition and Dietetics: The role of nutrition in health promotion and chronic disease prevention, *Journal of the Academy of Nutrition and Dietetics* 113 (2013): 972-979.

5. Whitney, Ellie, and Sharon Rady Rolfes. *Understanding Nutrition*. Cencage Learning, 2016.

6. Pollack, B. (2018). *phdeadlift.com | Unf*ck Your Warmup.* [online] Phdeadlift.teachable.com. Available at: https://phdeadlift.teachable.com/blog/1579095/uywarmup [Accessed 7 Aug. 2018].

7. Haddad, M, et al. "Static Stretching Can Impair Explosive Performance for at Least 24 Hours." *Advances in Pediatrics.*, U.S. National Library of Medicine, Jan. 2014, www.ncbi.nlm.nih.gov/pubmed/23615481.

8. Schoenfeld, B J, et al. "Effects of Low- vs. High-Load Resistance Training on Muscle Strength and Hypertrophy in Well-Trained Men." *Advances in Pediatrics.*, U.S. National Library of Medicine, Oct. 2015, www.ncbi.nlm.nih.gov/pubmed/25853914.

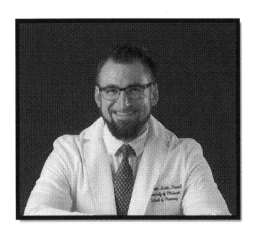

About the Author

Dr. Adam Martin earned his doctorate of pharmacy degree from the University of Pittsburgh School of Pharmacy. With over 7 years of experience working full-time in the community pharmacy setting, he's passionate about empowering other pharmacists and pharmacy students to put the health back into healthcare through leading by example in their professional practice to not only live their best lives, but to inspire others along the way to do the same. He is the founder of The Fit Pharmacist, a company with a mission to
empower stressed pharmacists with simple, effective plans to master their mindset, nail their nutrition, and fit fitness into their busy schedule. Through podcasting, collaborating with other passionate professionals across the profession, and delivering content across social media platforms such as LinkedIn, Facebook, and Instagram, The Fit Pharmacist strives to provide essential tools and resources enabling each and every member of our profession to make a difference in our patient's lives by starting with the source: YOU!

He currently resides in his hometown of Pittsburgh, PA, yet loves to travel the world with a passion for learning, serving, food-touring, and of course visiting innovative pharmacy schools and pharmacies along the way.

66855993R00044

Made in the USA
Middletown, DE
08 September 2019